Dolores Higgins
9971 Juniper Ave., Apt. 317
Fontana, CA 92335
(909) 233-5019


August 11, 2021


Woman's World Book Club
270 Sylvan Ave
Englewood Cliffs, NJ 07632


Enclosed is a copy of my book "Memories of Caring for my Aging Parents" (with Alzheimer's Disease). This book is also available on Amazon.

I am not sure if this is the type of material you seek for your Book Club, so if it isn't, if possible, would you return it to me? If you are not able to do that, I do understand.

Thank you for your consideration for the Book Club.

Sincerely,

Dolores Higgins

# Memories of Caring for my Aging Parents

## with Alzheimer's Disease

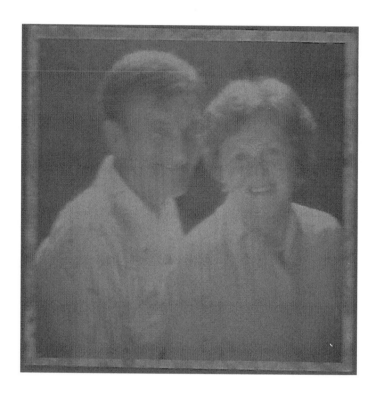

By

*Dolores M. Higgins*

# Introduction

For a total of 18 years, I was caregiver for my parents. The first ten I assisted my mother while she took care of my father. After my father passed my mother quickly declined. I then became her sole caregiver for the last eight years of her life.

Within these pages, are some of my personal experiences; my solutions to problems that arose; as well as, some funny stories while caring for both my parents with Alzheimer's.

The original plan was to record only the humorous events. However, my daughter, Shelly, encouraged me to record all incidences since this disease affects the whole family, not only the caregiver. I then included background information and research so readers can see the whole picture of what the disease is about, and what it's like taking care of someone with Alzheimer's, as well as, what to expect. I hope I have succeeded in conveying this to you, the reader.

# Table of Contents

# A Special Thanks

Although my parents are no longer with me, I want to express my gratitude here for the wonderful childhood that they gave me during war years and post-war years; (the late 30s into the early 1940s). Even though I am an only child, I was no way "spoiled." They taught me honesty, responsibility, gratitude, and appreciation for whatever I was given, in addition to how to be a hard worker, and a person of my word, and so many other old-fashioned characteristics. But I learned the most by their example. It was an honor to be able to care for them in their last years.

I want to also thank my youngest daughter, Shelly Thie, for her willingness to proof-read the books I attempt to write. She always has wise advice and catches my errors. And a special thank you Shelly, for your suggestion that I include the difficult times and not only the humorous events that I went through caring for my parents. It was you who said people need to know the difficulties that arise in a situation like this one.

*Dolores M. Higgins*

# Chapter 1

## EXACTLY WHAT IS ALZHEIMER'S?

If you are going to be a caregiver for a loved one with dementia or progressive Alzheimer's, it would be helpful to gather all the information and facts of these diseases so you are better prepared mentally and emotionally for the journey you are about to encounter.

Alzheimer's disease is an irreversible, progressive brain disorder that slowly destroys the memory and other important mental functions. Sometimes, it is diagnosed as, "mild cognitive impairment." Either way, eventually, the disease destroys one's ability to carry out simple everyday tasks. It is the most common cause of dementia in older adults. The formal definition is: *"Progressive mental deterioration that can occur in middle or old age, due to generalized degeneration of the brain. It is the most common cause of premature senility."*

Dementia is more common as people grow older; however, it is not a normal part of aging as some may believe, although age is the greatest risk factor.

Unfortunately the disease worsens over time. A person may have dementia but may not have Alzheimer's. But with Alzheimer's there is always dementia. The way Alzheimer's is diagnosed; is by ruling out the other questionable options.

Alzheimer's is the sixth leading cause of death in the United States so far with no cure. This disease is ranked third behind heart disease and cancer, mostly among the elderly. A person can live an average of eight years after the symptoms are noticeable although some can survive up to 20 years – depending on their age and health conditions.

## THE SEVEN (7) STAGES OF ALZHEIMERS:

So that you are better prepared you should be aware of the different stages of Alzheimer's. It will help you understand what to expect and possibly reduce some of your confusion.

Stage 1: No Impairment
Unfortunately, during this stage, Alzheimer's is not detectable and no memory problems or other symptoms of dementia are evident.

Stage 2: Very Mild Decline
The person may notice minor memory problems or lose things around the house, although not to the point where the memory loss can easily be distinguished from normal age-related memory loss. The person will still do well on memory tests and the disease is unlikely to be detected by loved ones or physicians.

Stage 3: Mild Decline
At this stage, the family members and friends of the person may begin to notice cognitive problems. Performance on memory tests are affected and physicians will be able to detect impaired cognitive function. People in Stage 3 will have difficulty in many areas including:
- Finding the right word during conversations or repeating themselves.
- Organizing and planning.
- Remembering names of new acquaintances.

People with Stage 3 Alzheimer's may also frequently lose personal possessions, including valuables.

Stage 4:  Moderate Decline:
In Stage 4 there are more clear-cut symptoms than with the first three stages. The symptoms of the disease are apparent. These symptoms are:
- Have difficulty with simple arithmetic.
- Have poor short-term memory (for example they may not recall what they ate for breakfast).
- Inability to manage finances and pay bills.
- May forget details about their life histories.

Stage 5:  Moderately Severe Decline:
During the fifth stage of Alzheimer's, people begin to need help with many day-to-day activities. People in Stage 5 may experience:
- Difficulty dressing appropriately.
- Inability to recall simple details about themselves such as their own phone number.
- Significant confusion.

On the other hand, people in Stage 5 maintain functionality. They typically can still bathe and toilet independently. They also usually still know their family members and some detail about their personal histories, especially their childhood and youth.

Stage 6:  Severe Decline:
People with the sixth stage of Alzheimer's need constant supervision and frequently require professional care. Symptoms include:
- Confusion or unawareness of environment and surroundings.
- Inability to recognize faces except for the closest friends and relatives.
- Inability to remember most details of personal history.
- Loss of bladder and bowel control.
- Major personality changes and potential behavior problems.

- The need for assistance with activities of daily living - such as toileting and bathing.
- Wandering.

Stage 7: Very Severe Decline:
Stage 7 is the final stage of Alzheimer's. Because the disease is a terminal illness, people in Stage 7 are nearing death. In Stage 7 of the disease, people lose the ability to communicate or respond to their environment. While they may still be able to utter words and phrases, they have no insight into their condition and need assistance with all activities of daily living. In the final stages of Alzheimer's, people may lose their ability to swallow.

It is easy to get concerned when you forget where you placed your keys or when you miss a bill payment. You may think, "I hope this is not the beginning of Alzheimer's disease." But often, this is just because of being too busy and nothing to be overly concerned about.

Here are some early signs of the disease as published by the National Institute on Aging:

1 – Cognitive memory decline that disrupts daily life.
2 – Challenges in planning or solving problems, inability to do simple math.
3 – Difficulty completing familiar tasks at home, work, or at leisure; i.e. paying bills or solving simple math problems.
4 – Confusion with time or place; not knowing the date or time of the year. Mental confusion, difficulty concentrating.
5 – Trouble understanding visual images and solid relationships.
6 – New problems with words in speaking or writing; difficulty having fluent conversations.
7 – Misplacing things and losing the ability to retrace steps.
8 – Decreased or poor judgment.
9 – Withdrawal from work or social activities.

10 - Changes in mood; anger, apathy, loneliness, or mood swings.
11 – Changes in personality. Behavioral changes such as aggression, agitation, irritability, wandering and getting lost.
12 – Psychological changes; depression, hallucination, or even paranoia.

In addition, here are some possible signs of normal aging:

1 - Making a bad decision on occasion.
2 - Missing one monthly bill payment.
3 - Sometimes forgetting which word to use.
4 - Occasionally losing some things, including your keys.

What should you do if you notice these signs in yourself or your loved one? First of all, do not ignore them. Schedule an appointment with the doctor. With early detection, you can explore treatments that may provide some relief of symptoms and help maintain a level of independence longer; as well as increase the chances of participating in clinical drug trials that help advance research.

When people with Alzheimer's disease and related disorders, behave in ways that a caregiver may interpret as challenging, they need to recognize that all behavior is a form of communication. The question to ask is - what the person is trying to communicate. It is important to recognize any new behaviors in the person.

When it comes to administering medication, it is not uncommon for a person with dementia or Alzheimer's to refuse. It may taste bad, or it may upset their stomach, or it may make them tired. And of course it could be that they just don't feel like taking any at that moment. Don't fuss with them. If they just "don't feel like it," this is considered resistant behavior. Find out what is triggering this resistance before trying to fix it.

For example, some Alzheimer's patients get distressed seeing a bottle filled with pills. If this might be the case, take the pills out of the bottle, and keep the bottle out of sight. If the size of the pills is the problem, check with the pharmacist and see if the pills come in a liquid form which would be easier to disguise in the food. Ask if they can be cut or crushed and put in the food. If the taste of the pill is the culprit, combine the pill with food that tastes good.

I personally faced this dilemma with my mother, she counted her pills each day so when the psychiatrist prescribed her two extra pills for her moods she refused to take them knowing she only took six pills, not eight. Rather than fuss with her, my solution was to crush the pills and insert them in the bottom of her favorite cookies. She always had two cookies after her meals. These cookies had a graham cracker bottom which was covered with chocolate. I crushed the pills, dug a little hole in the bottom of each cookie, put the pills inside, and covered it up with the chocolate. Wa-La! Problem solved! No more fuss, but most important, she was taking the pills that she needed. So there may be times you have to be a little creative in order to avoid a confrontation that would not be healthy for either one of you.

If taking care of a parent – or spouse - when you take into consideration all they have done for you, it can become a love journey, returning all the love they bestowed to you and others – back onto them with gratitude.

# Chapter 2

## A CAREGIVERS' DILEMMA

As is usually the case, my parents Alzheimer's started in their senior years, but I too was a senior. Being a caregiver for someone with Alzheimer's can be very stressful and many times takes a toll on the caregiver's health. There may even be times when you will feel "trapped" by Alzheimer's.

However, during the period of caring for a loved one with this disease there can also be some humorous events that take place that can sometimes outweigh the more challenging and stressful times. It was the amusing times that prompted me to write this book.

I lost my father in 1999 to this dreadful disease, and my mother in 2007. Being an only child I was the only one available to care for them. One thing I am most grateful for is that I was fortunate to be able to keep both of them at home until they breathed their last breath.

As mentioned, this disease is certainly not humorous, however there were times that made me smile over some of the incidences that happened and the comments that each of them would make. Yes there were times we could laugh as well as the times when we would cry; but I must add, the joyous and witty moments, truly did outweigh the bad. These are the times I remember and share with others the most.

To limit challenges you may face and ease your frustration, here are some useful suggestions:

1. – Schedule wisely. Establish a routine to make each day less agitating and confusing.
2. – Take your time. Expect things to take longer than they used to.
3. – Involve the person as much as you can.
4. – Provide choices. Leave some simple choices that they can make.
5. – Provide simple instruction when talking to them. Use few words so they can understand what you are asking of, or telling them.
6. – Reduce distractions. Distractions can confuse them, although sometimes necessary to get their mind off something.

Take into consideration any suggestions you may come across in literature. Do research on how you can make it easier on yourself. Be open to others' ideas and suggestions.

# Chapter 3

## BEGINNING OF A LONG JOURNEY

If you find me mentioning Opa within this book, I am referring to my father. The name Opa is German for grandfather, and Oma means grandmother. When my husband and I came back from Germany we decided to have our children call my parents Oma and Opa and ever since then, even our friends called them by those names.

Opa got Alzheimer's first. As is usually the case, like mentioned in the different stages, it sneaks up on you, especially if you are not familiar with the symptoms. Which my mother and I were not.

The day my father surrendered his driver's license was a surprise to my mother and me. We never thought he would ever, ever do that! We discovered later that when he would go out sometimes he could not remember how to get home. He had taken care of his father-in-law, Grandpa Anderson, years ago. They would talk of times when grandpa would go for a walk and get lost, not knowing how to get home. So I could only presume that my father knew he was having a serious problem when he got lost. For all we knew, he may have had some close calls that he never shared with any of us... we will never know for sure. But, he did surrender his license admitting that he was no longer capable of driving. That was just the beginning of our long journey down this new road of Alzheimer's.

Shortly after, his health slowly started to decline, as well as his mental aptitude. At first we thought it was his hearing. So my mother had his hearing aids checked. The doctor explained to her that it was not his hearing but rather (the doctor pointed to his own head) he said it was his thinking process.

Since it was not that prevalent during those years there was very little information available to us. We found ourselves learning as we went along.

Oma was Opa's primary caregiver. I merely helped her. She had asked me to come live with them. Little did I know at that time, my mother was having some minor mental difficulties of her own, which surfaced later.

Once we realized we were up against a more serious circumstance than we first anticipated, we brought it to the attention of my father's primary doctor who was very supportive and gave my father many tests. These tests confirmed what we feared my father did indeed have Alzheimer's.

My mother had a geriatric doctor along with her primary doctor. However with my father I don't recall there being a geriatric doctor available for him since he got the disease many years prior.

Opa was always an active man. He was also a very loving and compassionate man. He would always be there for anyone who needed assistance in any area that was required. However, he could be a very stubborn man as well. As the disease progressed, his personality changed, and he became more of a challenge.

Before been stricken with this disease he would putter around outside every day. He was a very resourceful person and would come up with ideas to make the landscape and the house look better. Then, after a few months, his activities became fewer and fewer. He stopped going outside to putter and begin to sit in his recliner and sleep more often.

As my father progressively declined and his health became more of a serious problem, his primary doctor advised my mother to have him put on hospice. The doctor explained he felt Opa had only a couple more months to live. Needless to say this news was devastating to my mother and myself. Opa was on hospice for approximately three months before he passed.

If you should have the option to put your loved one on hospice per your doctor's recommendation, I would strongly recommend this. Hospice was marvelous! They helped with bathing, medicines, would even come to visit so my mother could get out of the house while I was at work. My father loved reading and the volunteer would read to him. The hospice doctor kept us informed on a weekly basis of Opa's condition and prepared us with what to expect.

About two weeks before my father passed, the hospice doctor sat with my mother and I after he examined Opa. He discussed what we should expect for the next two weeks and he let us know that was about as long as my father was expected to survive.

After the doctor left ... my mother came into my room with tears in her eyes. She had done the math, just as I had, but I did not mention anything to her. I recall her standing at the door saying, "Dolores in two weeks that will be our 61st wedding anniversary and also Opa's birthday." I went to her, put my arms around her and said, "I know mom." And we had a good cry together.

One week went by and then we were starting into the second week. Opa's birthday was on the 8<sup>th</sup> of June and it was the same day my mother had a stroke. I always figured it was because of her anticipation of his passing being so close to his birthday and their anniversary coming up on the 11<sup>th</sup> and realizing this may be his last week with us. My father was in a coma during the time the paramedics took my mother to the hospital.

The next morning I was awakened with what they call the death rattle. I realized from the pamphlets hospice gave us, that my father was breathing his last breath. I have wondered, even though he was in the coma, he might have been aware of what was happening to her when the paramedics took her out of the bedroom. I'll never really quite know.

Let me add here ... the pamphlets, the advice and the counseling that we got from the hospice doctor and nurses made this transition so much easier. I did not say easy, I said it made it easier. I cannot thank the hospice staff enough for all their care and support.

# Chapter 4

## MY FATHER aka OPA

My father's father, my grandfather, who was white, married an Indian woman. He was murdered when my father was in eighth grade. They lived on an Indian reservation in Omaha, Nebraska. My father never talked about grandpa's murder but when his sister, (my Aunt Betty) came to visit us she gave me the details of what she knew.

My grandfather had a concession stand on the Pow Wow grounds of the Indian reservation. There was a Marshall that liked my grandmother and he and my grandfather got in an argument when they were at the Pow Wow grounds. The next day grandpa disappeared and was never seen again. The rumor that spread was that grandpa was murdered and his body thrown in the Missouri River. This was back in the early 1900s, with the suspect being the Marshall and my grandmother being an Indian, you didn't dare get involved or say anything.

My father was only in eighth grade at the time and the oldest son at home. The elder son Elmer was in the Army so my father had to quit school at eighth grade to take care of his siblings. Since his mother was American Indian they were able to stay on the reservation to live.

My father had very little education so he became a self-taught man. There really wasn't anything he could not do. He would check books out from the library and taught himself air conditioning, heating, auto mechanics, construction; you name it he could do it. He even started making his own electric car way before its time. His trade however was upholstery of which he was one of the best! I've heard it said that Indians are good with their hands and artistic. Maybe this is why Opa was such a good upholsterer.

At the beginning of my father's illness, he was easy to care for. At times he could be a lot more stubborn than my mother had been, and at times more difficult to handle. But, when I couldn't handle a situation my mother could, and vice versa. He was a good man and always worked hard to support his family. He was of the generation where the majority of the people were honest and had integrity. More than once he took in family members who were either ill and needed help or just a straying niece who needed family to care for her.

One day I came home from church and as I walked in the door my father was coming up the hallway with his walker. I could tell he was upset. Just as I came in the door he threw his walker across the room! He just barely missed the wall where we had mirror panels. This was really about the only time I saw him out of control but it was a little scary. Then he walked over and sat down in his recliner.

My mother came up the hall shortly after with tears in her eyes. She said shockingly, "Opa hit me in the mouth!" This was as much a surprise to her as it was to me. My father never, never hit my mother. Meanwhile Opa is sitting in his recliner and appeared to be totally oblivious to what he had just done.

Now I don't know if what I did next is the right thing to do or not... but I walked over and quietly and politely, but very firmly let him know what he did and he was to never do that again. I could tell by the way he looked at me he was shocked at himself. But I will say he never did it again.

My father was a very caring, kind, and thoughtful man and when he passed it was just two days before my parents' 61st wedding anniversary. He loved my mother immensely and she him.

Some may become more combative than others and may even break things. If this should happen please be sure to contact the doctor for assistance.

I cannot repeat this enough, but it is important that you remember they will go through many different mood swings and you will have to deal with them. If you can mentally and emotionally remember that and try your best to prepare for them, it will make your caregiving much easier.

# Chapter 5

## HERE WE GO AGAIN

With my mother having her stroke and in rehabilitation, I had to prepare the funeral plans for my father by myself. This was probably for the best because my mother was not in the frame of mind to do so even before her stroke. This also gave me time to have my father's hospital bed removed and put the bedroom back into its original state prior to his illness.

My mother's doctor said she could go to the viewing although he recommended against it for fear of her having another stroke. She took her doctor's advice and did not attend the viewing, but did attend the funeral. The mortician was kind enough to make it possible for her to see my father briefly before taken to the gravesite. This was important for her closure.

Shortly after the funeral my mother was able to come home. I was now her sole caregiver. She had a peaceful nature but sometimes her moods changed. Since I had been through this once before I knew to log some of the issues that came up and let her doctor know about them. He was able to prescribe medication that helped keep her calm. There were times when her moods would be combative but this was seldom. Basically she was pleasant to be around and easy to attend to. I was fortunate in that way.

As mentioned, the beginning of this terrible disease is sometimes difficult to spot. At first I wasn't sure if it was the stroke she had or the early stages of Alzheimer's. But soon I knew it was more than the stroke. There would be days when the mail lady would bring 2-3 buckets of mail a week to our door! Then, when bills went unpaid I knew there was something drastically wrong! My parents were very old-school they never let a bill go unpaid.  One day I finally had to approach my mother about this. That is when she broke down crying and said she had been meaning to ask me for help with the finances.

After reviewing her checking account, I discovered many more bills had gone unpaid and she was spending literally hundreds of dollars on charities that would send her two to four notices a month!  You must really watch out for duplicate notices from charities and the like. They take advantage of seniors and anytime she would send in a check they would send her another request, rather than wait a month to do so.

It was then I had to develop a serious plan on getting the important bills paid and up-to-date and then the most difficult of all, stop all the charity mailings in addition to those from Publisher Clearing House, Readers Digest, and the like. She would often order the same items 2-3 times from all of them and she kept them hidden in her bedroom chest, which I discovered later. Fortunately, as mentioned later, I was able to return several of the items and get her a refund.

Calling or writing to them telling them to stop got me nowhere. The only thing that worked was putting in a change of address and I had all her mail sent to my PO Box. I would not respond to the requests and instead threw away the mail as it came in. I was gradually able to stop the vultures that prey on declining seniors. But it took up to two years to finally stop all the "junk" mail.

I personally made a call to the headquarters office of Publishers Clearing House and to Readers Digest and was able to return around $2,000 of items to each company. So there was around $4,000 I was able to retrieve for my mother. But it definitely was not an easy task and was only a drop in the bucket of all the money my mother had sent to them. Going through this stress eventually affected my health, causing me blood pressure problems.

My mother was still able to drive her car on short runs like to the beauty parlor. She would pick up a friend and the two of them would go get their hair done. One day as she was pulling out from the side street after picking up her friend and she pulled out right in front of an oncoming car. Fortunately, my mother and her friend were not hurt nor were the two men in the other car. The two men in the other car were also very kind and thoughtful to my mother. The tow truck brought the car and my mother home and I took care of arrangements of having the car repaired and listening to my mother side of the story of what happened. We later discovered her car was totaled.

Her side, as far as she understood, and the way she relayed it to me, made sense. I had no reason to doubt it, but as it turned out her "memory" was not as she thought it was and she was 100% at fault. It was definitely a blessing that no one was hurt. I knew at this point something had to be done. My mother should not be behind the wheel of a car.

My mother started talking about buying another car. I could not allow to happen. But, what could I do to prevent it without causing a problem between us? Finally a solution came to my mind.

I wrote a letter to the DMV office (requesting complete confidentiality) informing them of my mother's accident, explaining that she was 100% at fault and let them know of her failing mental health. They sent a letter to her telling her she must come in for a behind the wheel test. When she read the letter she misinterpreted it as them telling her she could not drive anymore. I asked her if I could see the letter and I ended up putting it in the trash. There was no more mention from her of getting a car or driving. She had forgotten the whole matter.

Was this an inconvenience to me? Of course it was but it was the safest thing to do in the most loving thing to do for my mother and all those that on the road. By contacting DMV and them sending her a letter I was not the bad guy. My father willingly gave up his driver's license, but my mother was not about to do so willingly, even after her accident.

Just as I had to come up with a solution to prevent a serious problem, so you will have to be "on your toes. You must always be one step ahead of the game. This, in itself, is no easy task. But, rest assured, you will find a way around and over all the hurdles you face.

# Chapter 6

## SOME AMUSING MOMENTS

So far, I have shared with you some examples of the seriousness of this disease. Now I would like to tell you some humorous and cute stories. It's not all doom and gloom. At least for myself it was not. There was a good balance. In fact the times I remember the most and share with others are the cute little incidences that came up. As a caregiver you must learn to be flexible and you can never anticipate just what they are going to say or do. You will find the Alzheimer's patient can be a person of many moods and sometimes when you least expect it.

The story or I should say the memory that is one of the fondest I have of my mother is when I was in my room at my computer. My mother walks up the hall stands in the doorway and shakes her finger at me and says ...

"Dolores! Do you have your driver's license?"

In amazement I looked up at her and said, "Mom, I'm 67 years old. I've had my license since I was 16."

She gave me the most bewildered look and said questionably, "You're 67?" Then confidently she said ..."You're Dorothy."

Dorothy was her sister whom she got me confused with often. I said,

"No... I'm Dolores."

She wrinkled her brow and thought about it a bit then turned and walked back down the hall murmuring to herself ...    "I'm living with an old woman."

I sat there and laughing to myself. She was absolutely serious when she said that.

Another time was when my mother requested I do something for her. It was the way she asked that I thought was quite clever. She liked to sit in her rocking recliner, watching television and nibble on snacks and candy. She could also look out the front window and watch the neighbors or people walking by. Next to her chair was a round tin. For those of us who remember the button tins, it was like that. Oma kept candy in hers.

So one day she walks up to me, didn't say a word just smiled with her sweet little smile and handed me her round tin. She then turned and walked back to her room. When I open the tin there was a note inside that said, "Feed me." She wanted more candy. I chuckle every time I think of this incident.

So ... if you end up a caregiver please take the time to record your positive experiences. When your loved one is gone, you'll be glad you did. These will be the memories you want to reflect on the most.

Since my mother was my father's primary caregiver and I only helped her, I don't have as many stories about my father but there are a couple that come to mind.

My father had contracted some kind of infection and was admitted to the hospital. We could tell he was not doing well at all and at one point we thought we were going to lose him. In addition, he was getting despondent being there.

I got this grand idea to sneak their little poodle, Bitsy, into the hospital for my father. Well the day I decided to do it the weather was extremely hot in fact I recall vividly the temperature was 102° which is not uncommon for a summer day in Southern California.

I covered Bitsy with a pink baby blanket. A friend and I started walking towards the entrance of the hospital. Since I used to work there, I knew a back way so we could sneak the dog in. As we were heading towards the back entrance, a woman walked past us and critically said "Look at that woman, she has her baby all bundled up in that blanket!" My friend quickly turned to the woman and said, "It's HER baby..." We laughed as we rushed up the back stairs.

As we slipped up the back stairway, we hurried down the hall and into my father's room. I quickly set Bitsy on my father's chest. His eyes were closed but as soon as he felt his little furry friend on his chest he opened his eyes and gave us one of the biggest, toothless grins ever.

As fate would have it, a nurse walked in about that time. She informed us that they now allow therapy animals in the hospital and we really didn't have to sneak her in.

Looking back I think it was more fun sneaking the dog in..... Wouldn't you agree?

Another time when my father was in the hospital, the nurse relayed an incident she thought was kind of cute. She said Opa had tried to get out of bed and fell on the floor, belly-down. He was still connected to oxygen, IVs, and everything. As she walked by the room she looked in and when he saw her, he raised his arm up in the air and said, "Take me to your leader!" I guess he reverted back to World War II. We'll never know.

# Chapter 7

## FACING CHALLENGES
### (And You Will)

There will be times that will be more stressful than others. This is to be expected. One day a man from my church came to help with some handiwork. He brought along his teenage son. I was standing at the end of the hall discussing what needed done when my mother came storming up the hallway. This was one of her bad days. She put her hand out and demanded, very firmly. "Dolores! Give me my checkbook!"

As I've said before you never know what to expect, and you never know what kind of mood they might be in. The three of us stood there dumbfounded. I replied, "Mom, I can't. I am supposed to keep the checkbook."

She put her hand on her hip and looked at the man saying, "Hummmpf what do you think of a daughter who won't give her mother her own checkbook?"

Of course, the man and his son were speechless and just looked at one another. She turned and walked back down the hall. A few moments later, she didn't recall anything that had just transpired.

Not to be disrespectful to my mother, I know this was stressful for her, but it was a little humorous and we did get a little chuckle out of it once the shock wore off. Your life is going to be full of surprises and there will be times you will be totally unprepared. Just remember, this is part of the disease and don't take things personally their anger is not against you.

The man told me a few days later they were at home and his son needed money for some supplies. He walked up to his father and said with his hand outstretched, "Give me the checkbook," which became a little joke around their house. Again, not showing any disrespect, but sometimes we need to laugh at the more trying incidences. I think this is what helped me maintain my balance and possibly my sanity.

Of course there were some tearful times. Once was when my mother would come to me and be a little more assertive then she was at other times. It was usually over her checkbook or her car which she forgot she no longer had. Each time it was about the same way. When she would repeat particular situations, I could then almost predict what was coming next and be prepared.

Whenever she would demand her checkbook I would remind her the doctor wanted me to handle everything for her because she was no longer able to do so. She would start to argue and I would have to reprint the doctor's letter where he stated that I was to handle her affairs, since she was no longer capable of doing so. I only did this when it was absolutely necessary and it would eventually calm her down. I would hand her the copy which she would take to her room to read.

Shortly after, she would come back up the hall, stand in my doorway, with tears in her eyes. She would say, "Dolores, I am so sorry that I am such a burden to you." I would put my arms around her and let her know she was not a burden to me. I loved her and I wanted to care for her and then we would have a good cry together.

However, a few days later... she would forget what had happened and the same incident would repeat itself. She'd insist on having her checkbook. And again, I would print out another copy of the letter, and the ending was always the same... We would hug each other and cry together. This is why I ended up scanning the doctor's letter. I couldn't let her have the original to read. I lost count of how many times I had to print out that letter. And, interestingly, when she passed on, I never found the copies in her room. So, I'm guessing she just put each of them in the trash.

You see, you must understand the disease of Alzheimer's, they do not remember current events as well as they do their childhood memories. So we must not be alarmed if they repeat themselves or ask the same questions over and over. You must and I do repeat, you must have patience with your loved one. Don't say, "I already told you..." this will cause more frustration on their part as it reminds them of their shortcomings. Their anger and frustration is more against themselves – not you. Sometimes they know something is wrong with them, they just don't know what and don't remember the details of how they have acted.

# Chapter 8

## OUR LAST VACATION TOGETHER

Shortly after my father's death, his only living sibling contacted us. This was his sister Betty Ann who lived in Missouri. I had not seen my Aunt Betty in 53 years and she had never been to California. So I thought it would be nice to have her come visit us. I decided to take her and my mother on a week vacation to San Diego. My mother's stage of Alzheimer's was progressing rapidly and I realized we would not have much more quality time together.

I contacted a bed-and-breakfast close to Old Town in San Diego and rented the top suite and an old Victorian Inn. I totally forgot I had two senior women with me who would have to walk up those stairs! Since it was an old Victorian home converted into a bed-and-breakfast, there was no elevator. And of course, I also was a senior. But all-in-all, we all survived.

I had a full itinerary planned for the ladies and we had only one day with nothing to do but rest. I figured we would need one day to relax. I took the ladies on a Gondola ride with the mandolin player, chocolate covered strawberries, and a view of beautiful homes along the water. We enjoyed that immensely. I also planned for a trip on one of the water buses. I didn't tell the ladies that the bus could actually go in the water so that was quite a surprise to them. They enjoyed seeing the sea lions sunbathing.

When you do special things with your loved one, especially a trip, make it easy on yourself as well. You will have your hands full as it is, so things like taking a taxi instead of driving and trying to and parking, or renting a wheelchair save a lot of time and hassle.

On our return trip home, we met my youngest daughter Shelly who came down from 29 Palms to meet her Great Aunt Betty. That day we went to Knott's Berry Farm and enjoyed their famous chicken dinner. Before my Aunt Betty went back to Missouri, she also met Shelly's two daughters Destine' and Amanda her Great-Great Nieces. I'll say one thing we did a lot of eating that week.

The night before Aunt Betty was to go home I fixed supper at our house. My mother was sitting across the table from Aunt Betty and they were visiting while they were eating. Then out of the blue, my mother looked at Betty and said, "You look just like O.G.'s sister Betty Ann." Now, my father's name was Oren George but people called him O.G. for short. Aunt Betty, ... in amazement, especially after spending a week together and reminiscing about the old times started pointing her finger at herself and said kind of shockingly ... "I 'AM' BETTY ANN !"

So you never when they can remember or when they will forget and you never know what's going to come out of the mouth of your loved one. Be prepared for some humorous remarks and of course the less humorous.

Remember, they don't have much of a memory of current events. Most of them fade quickly. What they remember the most are their younger years. I was glad I had my Aunt Betty come out. It made both of their last days memorable. Shortly after Aunt Betty arrived home, she fell, tripping over her cat and broke her hip. She passed on about five months after she arrived home. My mother passed two months after Aunt Betty. I'm grateful for the photo album I made of the memories of their last vacation together ... of which I was a part.

# Chapter 9

## ON THE DECLINE

One day I came home from a short trip to the store. My mother was sitting on the back porch steps. This was the first time she was ever out of the house when I returned from shopping. She wasn't locked out, just sitting on the back steps. She did not know or remember if she had gone anywhere but I knew then I had to keep a closer eye on her. It was fortunate that she didn't wander off, which they are inclined to do towards the end.

She seemed to develop an infection so I took her to the hospital. She was there all afternoon and evening until about 10:00pm. The doctor on at that time wanted to send her home with a high fever. I absolutely refused so he told me I would have to wait until the next doctor came on shift, which I did. When the new doctor came on I insisted my mother be admitted and have tests. She was in the hospital three days. When she finally came home she was never the same. She was put on Home Health Care where a nurse came out about 3 times a week. She did have an infection which they gave her medicine for, but she gradually started failing. Looking back I believe her organs were starting to shut down which happens when they have Alzheimer's.

Shortly after her stay in the hospital, her primary doctor received a report from the ER. He then called me and suggested I have her put on Hospice. My father was on Hospice so I knew this was only done at the end of their life. I guess I was in denial and did not want to have her put on since it seemed so final. However, I was told by a Hospice nurse that if my mother got better they would put her back on Home Health. So I agreed. My mother was put on Hospice on a Tuesday, and the following Sunday she was gone, much quicker than my father while on Hospice, and much quicker than I was prepared for.

Taking care of my mother after my father had passed away, I could never be gone very long but at least I was able to get away to go to the store or go to church. However towards the end when I went to church I did have to have someone come in and be at the house even though I had put my mother to bed.

Some states have a law protecting the elders from being neglected and left alone when they are unable to care for themselves so check your state to see what the laws are regarding seniors and senior abuse. I am sure you want what's best for your loved one. But as my mother declined I knew I could not leave her alone even though she was sleeping.

I was so grateful to be able to care for both my parents at home until their final days. I did not want to put them in a nursing home and fortunately I did not have to. If it had become impossible for me to take care of them, I was prepared to do this but did not want to.

# Chapter 10

## WHAT ARE YOU TO DO?

I gave you information on Symptoms of Alzheimer's and the different Stages the person might go through. I also gave you illustrations of some of my personal experiences, good and bad.

When caring for someone with Alzheimer's you must learn to live with unpredictability. There is no getting around it. That's just the way it is. Where you could once read a person like a book, it now becomes more of a puzzle. There will be a range of different emotions that arise at different times and probably when and where you least expect it. Try not to lose your patience. Just do your best and understand this is not the person you once knew. They cannot help their moods. Often, they aren't even aware of what they are doing or saying. If they have an outburst, it's best if you stop what you are doing and simply re-direct their thoughts. Redirecting their thoughts or attention is much easier and less stressful than fussing with them.

One thing to take serious consideration for, is that a person with Alzheimer's does not like change. It confuses them and when they get confused they get agitated and of course take it out on you or the closest person to them at that particular time. This can end up being more of a challenge for you.

To make your life and theirs easier, try to create a calm and quiet environment for them, by planning a daily schedule and try to maintain it. Remember too many changes only confused them. If you can have soothing music playing in the background, this could be helpful. Or if they like to watch television you choose the programs for them. You know what they like. And most of them enjoy comedy or animal programs and of course, nothing dramatic, loud, or violent.

Since my mother no longer knew how to control the television remote, every morning I would review the daily programs and would pre-set them so that when one was over it would automatically switch to the next program that I knew would hold her interest. You see, towards the end, that is about all she did was sit and watch television so I had to make sure it would be entertainment that she would enjoy. She loved I Love Lucy and animal shows.

When communicating with the person please use short sentences. Too much explanation only confuses them. You should be very brief and to the point. Nothing like this:

"Sit over there and wait for me because we're going to the doctor's and I still have to get ready."

Never use long sentences like that.

Instead say, "Sit and wait for me here." Keep it short and to the point.

Also, learn what part of the day is the best for your loved one. They will have good days and they will have bad days as you will quickly discover. For some they do better in the morning. Others do better in the evening. Then maybe a half hour later they are very confused. If necessary, log their good days and their bad days, the good times and the bad times to see if they have a pattern you can work with. However, it can also vary so be prepared for some drastic changes.

With some Alzheimer's patients there is what is called "sun-downing syndrome." This is a symptom of Alzheimer's and some other forms of dementia. It is also known as "late day confusion," which gets worse late in the afternoon or early evening. Fading light also seems to be a trigger to this. Stick to a daily routine and turn on the lights inside before it gets dark.

If you have difficulty getting them to take their medications try offering a reward, a favorite piece of candy might do the trick. Or do as I did by crushing the pill and inserting it in the bottom of a cookie.

And of course, it goes without saying that if you begin to notice additional changes with your loved one, please be sure to discuss this behavior with the doctor.

Do not be afraid or hesitant to ask for help. Whether it be through the doctor, or Hospice, and/or a family member. You must also take care of yourself. See that you can arrange a day off to take care of "your" needs. You can only be a good caregiver, if you care for yourself first.

# Chapter II

## THE ALZHEMER'S ASSOCIATION

If you are beginning to feel overwhelmed, by all means, seek support. There is no shame in seeking help. There are others who have been through the same predicament as you and many who are still going through it. There are many support groups to choose from and there is a lot of literature to read to better aid you in your journey.

The Alzheimer's Association has many pamphlets that will be helpful for caring for your loved one. As well as, for you, the caregiver. They can give you information on day care programs that may be available in your area.

The Alzheimer's Association also has information on what to expect in the last days. You need to be prepared for this also. Things like when to feed them or give them water and when not to. Feeding the patient towards the end could cause them to choke to death, which is much more drastic death than a natural, peaceful death. The Hospice doctor will most likely explain all of this when the time comes. Ours did and it was most helpful because it's natural to want to give them water or food. But there comes a time, when this can be fatal. So be sure to talk to the Hospice doctor and take heed to their advice.

The Alzheimer's Association teaches a three-step approach to understanding and adjusting to the behavior symptoms of Alzheimer's disease and related this orders. It is called IDEA.

'ID" - Identify the behavior. In some cases it may be their refusal to take medication.

"E" - Explore alternative reasons for the behavior. Is it new? Are they tired or irritable?

"A" - Adjust your approach. Try new strategies. Brainstorm. Remember, every person is different. Use trial and error to find an approach that works for you.

Being a caregiver for an Alzheimer's patient can be a long, lonely journey. However, it does not have to be that way. Today, there are more support groups and websites with an answer to any question you may have. They're available so use them.

Help you may find can apply to administering medication or simple tasks that your loved one is fighting against. Here are some helpful links:


**www.Alzgla.org/CaregiverTipSheets**
(for general tips and where to find a caregiver)

**www.Alz.org**
(for support groups & suggestions)

**www.AbesGarden.org**
(to watch videos offering caregiver tips
Plus they also have a newsletter available)


There are numerous tools that are available to you to make your journey smoother.

Some additional questions to ask yourself are:

- Is your loved one a danger to themselves?
- Does your love one present a danger to others?

As long as they are not in danger to themselves or others, you can let them make some of their own choices – within reason. At some point you need to except limits on what you can - or cannot - accomplish with your loved one. Do not feel "guilty" that you were having some difficulties. This is very normal in this kind of environment. And always have an "open door" of communication with your loved ones physician.

A question that may often come to your mind is... Will I also acquire Alzheimer's? After all they do is say it is hereditary. We read that genetic vulnerability and age is considered a risk factor for Alzheimer's disease. However, please be assured that having a parent with the disease is no guarantee that you will also have it.

There are many myths and misconceptions about Alzheimer's disease. What it is, who gets it, how it affects the people who have it, and what causes it. These myths stand in the way of fully understanding the disease and helping those who become affected. There are also many things that can help prevent it or delay onset. Such as a healthy diet, exercise, and avoiding head injuries, if possible.

Some feel aging can bring on Alzheimer's. This is not necessarily true. You may experience trouble with your memory as you age, which can be normal. However, if you notice that memory loss affects your day-to-day ability to do your regular routine, to function as normal, or to communicate properly, and of course, is accompanied by a decrease in judgment or reasoning ability, then it is best to see your doctor immediately for an evaluation.

The following was in a September 17, 2018, newspaper article "Successful Aging," by Helen Dennis. I felt it worthy to quote here. It's regarding the **"Best shield against Alzheimer's is ... LIFESTYLE."** As she stated, Scientists don't fully understand what causes Alzheimer's Disease. But, here is what they do know:

A genetic component plays a role for those who begin to get the disease in their 30s through mid-60s, affecting less than 10 percent of the cases. This is considered early onset. Late-onset the most common form, generally affects people older than 65 and likely is due to a complex series of brain changes occurring over decades that include genetic, environmental and lifestyle factors, according to the National Institute on Aging. Additional possible causes include inflammation in the brain and vascular risk factors. There is no known cure.

A little background:  The disease is named after Dr. Alois Alzheimer. In 1906, he noticed changes in the brain tissue of a woman who had died of an unusual mental illness characterized by memory loss, language problems and unpredictable behavior

After she died, he examined her brain and found abnormal clumps (now called amyloid plaques), and tangled bundles of fibers called tau or tangles.

Plaques and tangles are still considered main features of the disease, as is loss of connection between neurons.

These are nerve cells that transmit messages between different parts of the brain and from the brain to muscles and organs in the body. Scientists indicate that it is likely that damage to the brain starts about a decade before symptoms of memory loss and cognitive change become noticeable.

PREVENTION (to the extent possible) can be summed up in two words:  HEALTHY HABITS. Add to that a little luck, and still that is no guarantee.

The Harvard Health Letter (January 2017) recommends the following healthy habits:

**EXERCISE:** A review by scientists at the University of Southern California found that as many as 1 in 3 cases of Alzheimer's were preventable through lifestyle changes. One was physical exercise. The World Health Organization recommends that people 65 or older engage in 150 minutes of moderate aerobic exercise every week. Regarding vigorous aerobic exercise, WHO recommends 75 minutes a week. Add to that muscle-strengthening activity. The National Institute on Aging finds convincing evidence that physical exercise helps prevent the development of Alzheimer's or slows the progression in people who have symptoms. Regardless, we have everything to gain and nothing to lose, so get moving.

**EAT A MEDITERRANEAN DIET:** This has been shown to help prevent Alzheimer's or slow its progression. Partial adherence to such a diet is better than nothing. The diet includes fresh vegetables and fruits; whole grains; olive oil, nuts; legumes; fish; a moderate amount of poultry, eggs, and dairy; as well as a sparing amount of red meat.

**GET ENOUGH SLEEP:** Growing evidence suggests that improved sleep can help prevent Alzheimer's and is linked to greater amyioid clearance from the brain," says Dr. Gad Marshall of the Center for Alzheimer Research and Treatment at Harvard-affiliated Brigham and Women's Hospital. Aim for seven to eight hours per night.

**Other research indicates** the importance of stress management, learning new things and being socially engaged.

Although the research may not be conclusive, integrating these lifestyles into our daily lives can only serve us well. So, … let's all give it a try.

# Conclusion

I truly hope the contents within this book have been helpful to you. You are headed down a new road, a new experience, but you are not alone in this journey. There is more information available every day. Take advantage of the resources that are out there so you can prepare yourself.

If you find yourself at the beginning of this new road of caring for a loved one, just remember to be patient, log your fun times together so that when they are gone from your sight, you can remember the pleasant moments you had with them. These are the times you will want to focus on. There will be difficult and trying times but also cute and funny experiences.

I hope the contents in this book have been helpful to you and of some benefit as you and your love one begin your new walk down a new memory lane.

Most important of all, as you guide and direct your loved one think of it as a ... "Journey of the Heart."

And so, may your journey begin.

# About the Author

Dolores M. Higgins does not profess herself to be a writer. She writes when she is inspired and to record personal events for her family. For over 30 years she has dabbled in writing poetry, short stories, plays, children's stories, and even a movie script, which she anticipates someday converting into a novel. She received a First Place trophy for one of her short stories, and Second Place recognition on another, when she was a member of the Pomona Valley Writing Club. When they published a book in 1986, *"Expressions of the Soul ..."* a couple of her poems were included.  In addition, she enjoys baking and cooking so she put her favorite recipes into a cookbook as a special gift for her granddaughters.

It was not until recently, she learned how easily she could put her writings into print, if only as a keepsake for her children, grandchildren, great-grandchildren, and friends. It is her expectation to be able to put several more books in print after this one is completed.

Dolores was inspired to write this book about her personal experience in caring for her parents, who both ended up with Alzheimer's disease. It is her hope that her personal stories, information, and resources provided are helpful to others who may be faced with this same responsibility.

# Books  Available  by
# Dolores M. Higgins

"Prepare Your Own Living Trust,"  under  D.M. Higgins

"Total Health in a Nutshell"

"Spiritual Reflections"

"Memories of Caring for My Aging Parents"
(with Alzheimer's Disease)

"Mother, Grandma, Great-Grandma"   [ My story growing up ]
(Written mostly for my children)

# Books  Soon to Come by
# Dolores M. Higgins

"Eyes of the Beholder"

A Mother's Memoirs

The Other Side of the Bottle


And hopefully – many more

Books available at:  Amazon.com   ~and~   CreateSpace.com

Made in the USA
Middletown, DE
29 December 2020

30121955R10033